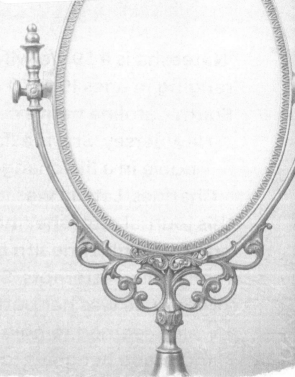

Journey to Wellness

Nateesha Blunt

About the Author

Nateesha is a 39 y/o wife and mother of 4 ranging in ages 19 to 10. She is a Columbia South Carolina native currently residing in New Jersey. She is a licensed practical nurse in a life changer for total Life Changes. Leticia was inspired to create this journal after she finally was successful and getting her health back on track after many failed attempts. She recognized the difference was her putting pen to paper which seemed to hold her accountable and made her goals towards becoming the best version of herself more realistic. Her hopes is for you to write down your dreams and your goals towards becoming the better version of you and see them unfold right before your eyes.

"journaling is paying attention to the inside for the purpose of living well from the inside out"
Lee Wise

My Daily Affirmations

I am peace
I am love
I am hope
I am wealthy
I am truth
I am strong
I am consistent
I am certain
I am fearless
I am happy
I am life
I am constant
I am blessed
I am wisdom
I am protected
I am limitless potential
I am one with the universe
I am positive
I am powerful

"If you can't be changed, you can't be alive. "

– James Baldwin

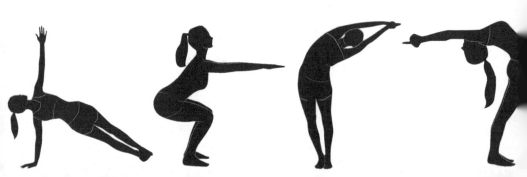

Reflection

date:

_____
_____
_____
_____
_____
_____
_____
_____
_____
_____
_____
_____
_____
_____
_____
_____
_____
_____
_____
_____
_____

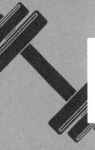

WORK IT!

WORKOUT PLANNER

	ACTIVITY	TIME	REPS
DAY 1	• Stretching & warm-up • Tempo-run 3 miles • Chest and shoulders	20 min 1,.5 hrs 2 hrs.	5 times 1 round 20 reps
DAY 2	• Legs and cardio • Easy run 3 miles • Wall Tricep Pushes	1 hr 30 mins 1.5 hrs	30 reps 1 round 50 reps
DAY 3	• Stretching & warm-up • Tempo-run 3 miles • Chest and shoulders	20 min 1,.5 hrs 2 hrs.	5 times 1 round 20 reps
DAY 4	• Legs and cardio • Easy run 3 miles • Wall Tricep Pushes	1 hr 30 mins 1.5 hrs	30 reps 1 round 50 reps
DAY 5	• Stretching & warm-up • Tempo-run 3 miles • Chest and shoulders	20 min 1,.5 hrs 2 hrs.	5 times 1 round 20 reps

WEEKLY FITNESS TRACKER

	DURATION	ACTIVITY
S		
M		
T		
W		
TH		
F		
S		

List Your #1 Goal

When do you think it will be completed?

Did you accomplish this goal?

Weekly Goal Planner

The Goal:

The Strategy:

Steps to Take:

Other Notes

Reflection

date:

_____

_____

_____

_____

_____

_____

_____

_____

_____

_____

_____

_____

_____

_____

_____

_____

_____

_____

AFFIRMATIONS

I am

MON
_____
_____

TUE
_____
_____

WED
_____
_____

THU
_____
_____

FRI
_____
_____

SAT
_____
_____

SUN
_____
_____

DATE

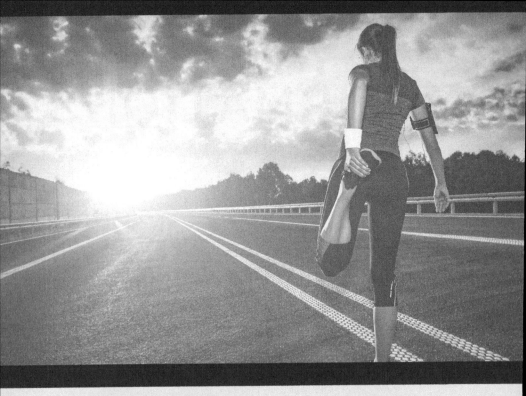

" ——————
Slow Progress
is better than
no progress
————— "

Reflection

date:

_____

_____

_____

_____

_____

_____

_____

_____

_____

_____

_____

_____

_____

_____

_____

_____

_____

_____

_____

_____

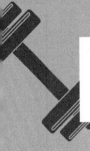

WORK IT!

WORKOUT PLANNER

	ACTIVITY	TIME	REPS
DAY 1	• Stretching & warm-up • Tempo-run 3 miles • Chest and shoulders	20 min 1,.5 hrs 2 hrs.	5 times 1 round 20 reps
DAY 2	• Legs and cardio • Easy run 3 miles • Wall Tricep Pushes	1 hr 30 mins 1.5 hrs	30 reps 1 round 50 reps
DAY 3	• Stretching & warm-up • Tempo-run 3 miles • Chest and shoulders	20 min 1,.5 hrs 2 hrs.	5 times 1 round 20 reps
DAY 4	• Legs and cardio • Easy run 3 miles • Wall Tricep Pushes	1 hr 30 mins 1.5 hrs	30 reps 1 round 50 reps
DAY 5	• Stretching & warm-up • Tempo-run 3 miles • Chest and shoulders	20 min 1,.5 hrs 2 hrs.	5 times 1 round 20 reps

WEEKLY FITNESS TRACKER

	DATE
	CURRENT WEIGHT

	DURATION	ACTIVITY
S		
M		
T		
W		
TH		
F		
S		

List Pain Points

When did it start?

What can you do to change it?

Reflection

date:

_____

_____

_____

_____

_____

_____

_____

_____

_____

_____

_____

_____

_____

_____

_____

_____

_____

_____

_____

_____

_____

Weekly Goal Planner

The Goal:

The Strategy:

Steps to Take:

- [ ]
- [ ]
- [ ]
- [ ]
- [ ]
- [ ]

Other Notes

WEEKLY
AFFIRMATIONS

I am

MON _____
_____

TUE _____
_____

WED _____
_____

THU _____
_____

FRI _____
_____

SAT _____
_____

SUN _____
_____

DATE

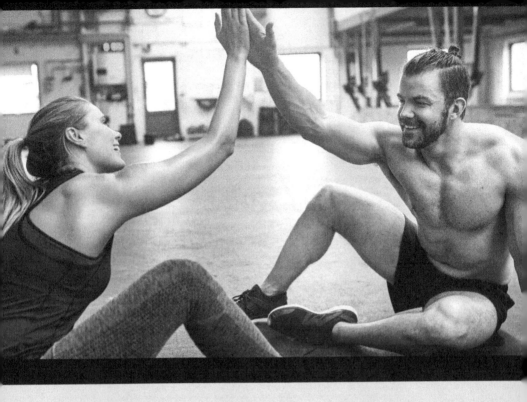

"
——————

A goal
is a dream
with a deadline

——————
"

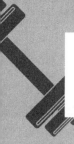
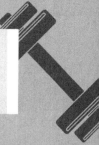

WORK IT!

WORKOUT PLANNER

	ACTIVITY	TIME	REPS
DAY 1	• Stretching & warm-up • Tempo-run 3 miles • Chest and shoulders	20 min 1,.5 hrs 2 hrs.	5 times 1 round 20 reps
DAY 2	• Legs and cardio • Easy run 3 miles • Wall Tricep Pushes	1 hr 30 mins 1.5 hrs	30 reps 1 round 50 reps
DAY 3	• Stretching & warm-up • Tempo-run 3 miles • Chest and shoulders	20 min 1,.5 hrs 2 hrs.	5 times 1 round 20 reps
DAY 4	• Legs and cardio • Easy run 3 miles • Wall Tricep Pushes	1 hr 30 mins 1.5 hrs	30 reps 1 round 50 reps
DAY 5	• Stretching & warm-up • Tempo-run 3 miles • Chest and shoulders	20 min 1,.5 hrs 2 hrs.	5 times 1 round 20 reps

WEEKLY FITNESS TRACKER

DATE

CURRENT WEIGHT

	DURATION	ACTIVITY
S		
M		
T		
W		
TH		
F		
S		

WEEKLY
AFFIRMATIONS

I am

MON
_____
_____

TUE
_____
_____

WED
_____
_____

THU
_____
_____

FRI
_____
_____

SAT
_____
_____

SUN
_____
_____

DATE

Reflection

date:

_____

_____

_____

_____

_____

_____

_____

_____

_____

_____

_____

_____

_____

_____

_____

_____

_____

_____

_____

"Pain will teach you things pride won't allow you to learn."

- Stormy Wellington

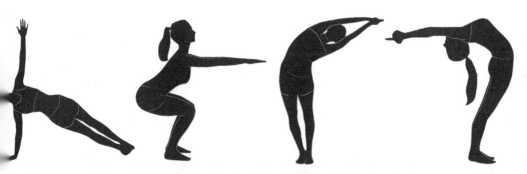

Weekly Goal Planner

The Goal:

The Strategy:

Steps to Take:

-
-
-
-
-
-

Other Notes

What goal didn't you accomplish?

How do you feel about it?

What can you do differently this week?

Reflection

_____

_____

_____

_____

_____

_____

_____

_____

_____

_____

_____

_____

_____

_____

_____

_____

_____

_____

_____

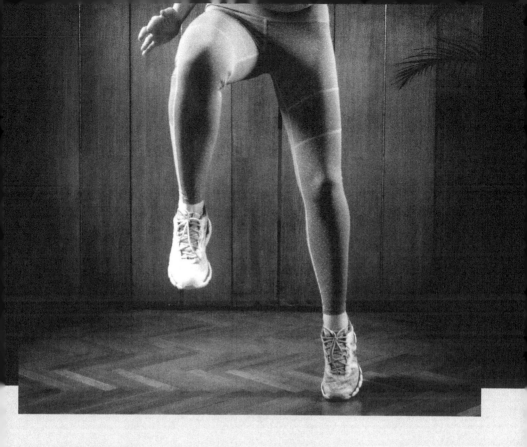

"—————

Respect your body
you only get one

—————"

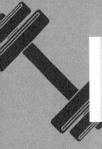

WORK IT!

WORKOUT PLANNER

ACTIVITY	TIME	REPS
DAY 1 • Stretching & warm-up • Tempo-run 3 miles • Chest and shoulders	20 min 1,.5 hrs 2 hrs.	5 times 1 round 20 reps
DAY 2 • Legs and cardio • Easy run 3 miles • Wall Tricep Pushes	1 hr 30 mins 1.5 hrs	30 reps 1 round 50 reps
DAY 3 • Stretching & warm-up • Tempo-run 3 miles • Chest and shoulders	20 min 1,.5 hrs 2 hrs.	5 times 1 round 20 reps
DAY 4 • Legs and cardio • Easy run 3 miles • Wall Tricep Pushes	1 hr 30 mins 1.5 hrs	30 reps 1 round 50 reps
DAY 5 • Stretching & warm-up • Tempo-run 3 miles • Chest and shoulders	20 min 1,.5 hrs 2 hrs.	5 times 1 round 20 reps

WEEKLY FITNESS TRACKER

DATE

CURRENT WEIGHT

	DURATION	ACTIVITY
S		
M		
T		
W		
TH		
F		
S		

AFFIRMATIONS

I am

MON
_____
_____

TUE
_____
_____

WED
_____
_____

THU
_____
_____

FRI
_____
_____

SAT
_____
_____

SUN
_____
_____

DATE

Nothing I ever want to accomplish will ever become a reality if I always quit.

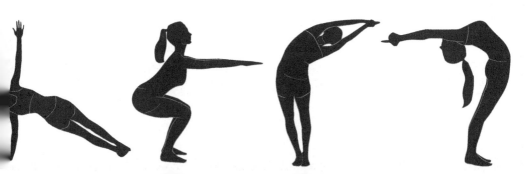

Weekly Goal Planner

The Goal:

The Strategy:

Steps to Take:

- [ ]
- [ ]
- [ ]
- [ ]
- [ ]
- [ ]

Other Notes

List Your #2 Goal

When do you think it will be completed?

Did you accomplish this goal?

Reflection

date:

_____

_____

_____

_____

_____

_____

_____

_____

_____

_____

_____

_____

_____

_____

_____

_____

_____

_____

_____

_____

Reflection

date:

Workout

> "Your body can almost stand anything"

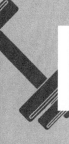

WORK IT!

WORKOUT PLANNER

ACTIVITY	TIME	REPS
DAY 1 • Stretching & warm-up • Tempo-run 3 miles • Chest and shoulders	20 min 1,.5 hrs 2 hrs.	5 times 1 round 20 reps
DAY 2 • Legs and cardio • Easy run 3 miles • Wall Tricep Pushes	1 hr 30 mins 1.5 hrs	30 reps 1 round 50 reps
DAY 3 • Stretching & warm-up • Tempo-run 3 miles • Chest and shoulders	20 min 1,.5 hrs 2 hrs.	5 times 1 round 20 reps
DAY 4 • Legs and cardio • Easy run 3 miles • Wall Tricep Pushes	1 hr 30 mins 1.5 hrs	30 reps 1 round 50 reps
DAY 5 • Stretching & warm-up • Tempo-run 3 miles • Chest and shoulders	20 min 1,.5 hrs 2 hrs.	5 times 1 round 20 reps

WEEKLY FITNESS TRACKER

DATE

CURRENT WEIGHT

	DURATION	ACTIVITY
S		
M		
T		
W		
TH		
F		
S		

AFFIRMATIONS

I am

MON
_____
_____

TUE
_____
_____

WED
_____
_____

THU
_____
_____

FRI
_____
_____

SAT
_____
_____

SUN
_____
_____

DATE

Reflection

date:

_____
_____
_____
_____
_____
_____
_____
_____
_____
_____
_____
_____
_____
_____
_____
_____
_____
_____
_____
_____

Suffer the pain of discipline or suffer the pain of regret.

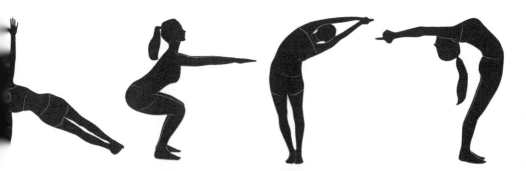

Weekly Goal Planner

The Goal:

The Strategy:

Steps to Take:

- [ ]
- [ ]
- [ ]
- [ ]
- [ ]
- [ ]

Other Notes

What goal didn't you accomplish?

How do you feel about it?

What can you do differently this week?

Reflection

date:

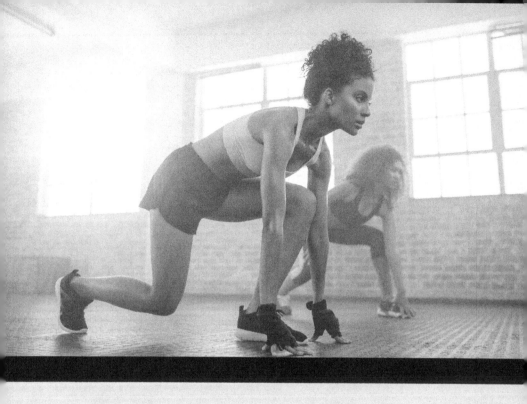

"

Think about why you started

"

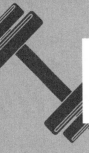

WORK IT!

WORKOUT PLANNER

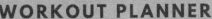

	ACTIVITY	TIME	REPS
DAY 1	• Stretching & warm-up • Tempo-run 3 miles • Chest and shoulders	20 min 1,.5 hrs 2 hrs.	5 times 1 round 20 reps
DAY 2	• Legs and cardio • Easy run 3 miles • Wall Tricep Pushes	1 hr 30 mins 1.5 hrs	30 reps 1 round 50 reps
DAY 3	• Stretching & warm-up • Tempo-run 3 miles • Chest and shoulders	20 min 1,.5 hrs 2 hrs.	5 times 1 round 20 reps
DAY 4	• Legs and cardio • Easy run 3 miles • Wall Tricep Pushes	1 hr 30 mins 1.5 hrs	30 reps 1 round 50 reps
DAY 5	• Stretching & warm-up • Tempo-run 3 miles • Chest and shoulders	20 min 1,.5 hrs 2 hrs.	5 times 1 round 20 reps

WEEKLY FITNESS TRACKER

DATE

CURRENT WEIGHT

	DURATION	ACTIVITY
S		
M		
T		
W		
TH		
F		
S		

AFFIRMATIONS

I am

MON
_____
_____

TUE
_____
_____

WED
_____
_____

THU
_____
_____

FRI
_____
_____

SAT
_____
_____

SUN
_____
_____

DATE

Reflection

date:

_____
_____
_____
_____
_____
_____
_____
_____
_____
_____
_____
_____
_____
_____
_____
_____
_____
_____
_____
_____
_____

Don't ask what the world needs ask what makes you come alive and go do it because what the world needs is more people who have come alive.

– Howard Thurman

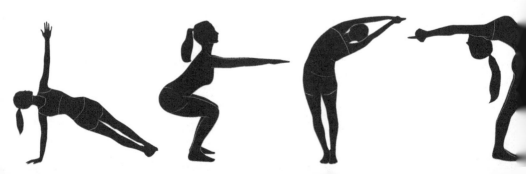

Weekly Goal Planner

The Goal:

The Strategy:

Steps to Take:

Other Notes

List Pain Points

When did it start?

What can you do to change it?

Reflection

date:

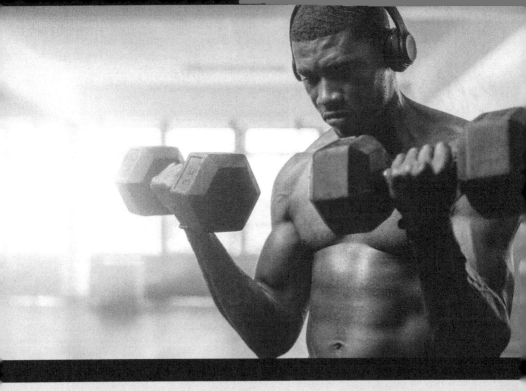

" —

Today's actions are tomorrow's results

— "

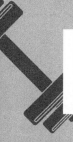

WORK IT!

WORKOUT PLANNER

	ACTIVITY	TIME	REPS
DAY 1	• Stretching & warm-up • Tempo-run 3 miles • Chest and shoulders	20 min 1,.5 hrs 2 hrs.	5 times 1 round 20 reps
DAY 2	• Legs and cardio • Easy run 3 miles • Wall Tricep Pushes	1 hr 30 mins 1.5 hrs	30 reps 1 round 50 reps
DAY 3	• Stretching & warm-up • Tempo-run 3 miles • Chest and shoulders	20 min 1,.5 hrs 2 hrs.	5 times 1 round 20 reps
DAY 4	• Legs and cardio • Easy run 3 miles • Wall Tricep Pushes	1 hr 30 mins 1.5 hrs	30 reps 1 round 50 reps
DAY 5	• Stretching & warm-up • Tempo-run 3 miles • Chest and shoulders	20 min 1,.5 hrs 2 hrs.	5 times 1 round 20 reps

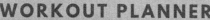

WEEKLY FITNESS TRACKER

CURRENT WEIGHT

	DURATION	ACTIVITY
S		
M		
T		
W		
TH		
F		
S		

AFFIRMATIONS

I am

MON
_____
_____

TUE
_____
_____

WED
_____
_____

THU
_____
_____

FRI
_____
_____

SAT
_____
_____

SUN
_____
_____

DATE _____

Personal development is the belief that you are worth the effort time and energy needed to develop yourself.

– Denis Waitley

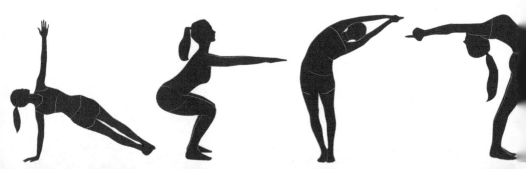

Weekly Goal Planner

The Goal:

The Strategy:

Steps to Take:

Other Notes

List Your #3 Goal

When do you think it will be completed?

Did you accomplish this goal?

Reflection

date:

_____
_____
_____
_____
_____
_____
_____
_____
_____
_____
_____
_____
_____
_____
_____
_____
_____
_____
_____
_____
_____

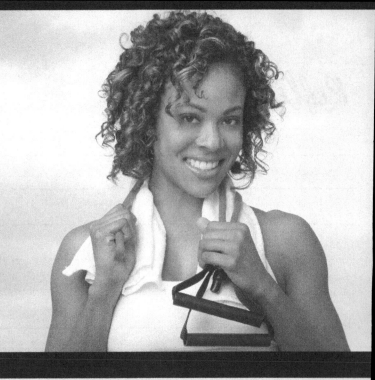

" ———

Don't STOP until you're

PROUD

——— "

WORK IT!

WORKOUT PLANNER

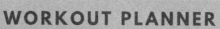

	ACTIVITY	TIME	REPS
DAY 1	• Stretching & warm-up • Tempo-run 3 miles • Chest and shoulders	20 min 1,.5 hrs 2 hrs.	5 times 1 round 20 reps
DAY 2	• Legs and cardio • Easy run 3 miles • Wall Tricep Pushes	1 hr 30 mins 1.5 hrs	30 reps 1 round 50 reps
DAY 3	• Stretching & warm-up • Tempo-run 3 miles • Chest and shoulders	20 min 1,.5 hrs 2 hrs.	5 times 1 round 20 reps
DAY 4	• Legs and cardio • Easy run 3 miles • Wall Tricep Pushes	1 hr 30 mins 1.5 hrs	30 reps 1 round 50 reps
DAY 5	• Stretching & warm-up • Tempo-run 3 miles • Chest and shoulders	20 min 1,.5 hrs 2 hrs.	5 times 1 round 20 reps

WEEKLY FITNESS TRACKER

DATE

CURRENT WEIGH

	DURATION	ACTIVITY
S		
M		
T		
W		
TH		
F		
S		

WEEKLY
AFFIRMATIONS

I am

MON _____
    _____

TUE _____
    _____

WED _____
    _____

THU _____
    _____

FRI _____
    _____

SAT _____
    _____

SUN _____
    _____

DATE _____

Reflection

date:

What we fear doing most is usually what we most need to do.

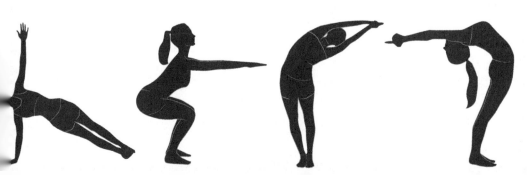

Weekly Goal Planner

The Goal:

The Strategy:

Steps to Take:

-
-
-
-
-
-

Other Notes

What goal didn't you accomplish?

How do you feel about it?

What can you do differently this week?

Reflection

date:

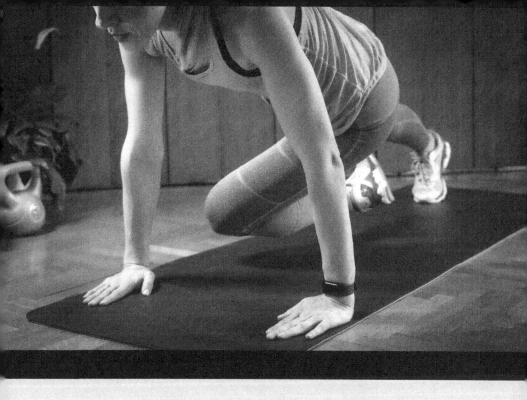

"

Sweat is just
Fat leaving
the body

"

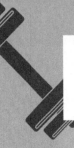

WORK IT!

WORKOUT PLANNER

ACTIVITY	TIME	REPS
DAY 1		
• Stretching & warm-up	20 min	5 times
• Tempo-run 3 miles	1,.5 hrs	1 round
• Chest and shoulders	2 hrs.	20 reps
DAY 2		
• Legs and cardio	1 hr	30 reps
• Easy run 3 miles	30 mins	1 round
• Wall Tricep Pushes	1.5 hrs	50 reps
DAY 3		
• Stretching & warm-up	20 min	5 times
• Tempo-run 3 miles	1,.5 hrs	1 round
• Chest and shoulders	2 hrs.	20 reps
DAY 4		
• Legs and cardio	1 hr	30 reps
• Easy run 3 miles	30 mins	1 round
• Wall Tricep Pushes	1.5 hrs	50 reps
DAY 5		
• Stretching & warm-up	20 min	5 times
• Tempo-run 3 miles	1,.5 hrs	1 round
• Chest and shoulders	2 hrs.	20 reps

WEEKLY FITNESS TRACKER

DATE

CURRENT WEIGHT

	DURATION	ACTIVITY
S		
M		
T		
W		
TH		
F		
S		

WEEKLY
AFFIRMATIONS

I am

MON _____
_____

TUE _____
_____

WED _____
_____

THU _____
_____

FRI _____
_____

SAT _____
_____

SUN _____
_____

DATE _____

Reflection

date:

_____
_____
_____
_____
_____
_____
_____
_____
_____
_____
_____
_____
_____
_____
_____
_____
_____
_____
_____

Weekly Goal Planner

The Goal:

The Strategy:

Steps to Take:

-
-
-
-
-
-

Other Notes

The struggle you're in today is developing the strength you need for tomorrow.

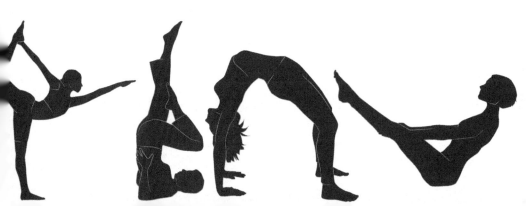

List Pain Points

When did it start?

What can you do to change it?

Reflection

date:

_____
_____
_____
_____
_____
_____
_____
_____
_____
_____
_____
_____
_____
_____
_____
_____
_____
_____
_____
_____
_____

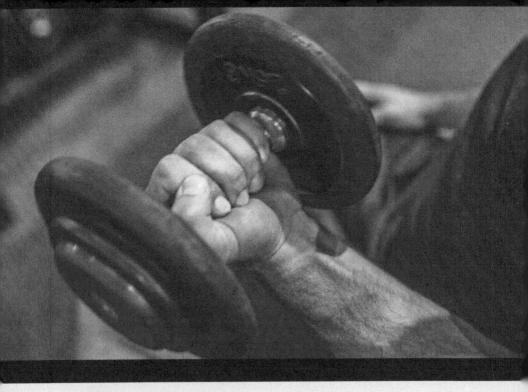

" ——————

No pain no gain
shut up and train

————— "

Reflection

date:

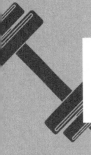

WORK IT!

WORKOUT PLANNER

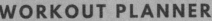

	ACTIVITY	TIME	REPS
DAY 1	• Stretching & warm-up • Tempo-run 3 miles • Chest and shoulders	20 min 1,.5 hrs 2 hrs.	5 times 1 round 20 reps
DAY 2	• Legs and cardio • Easy run 3 miles • Wall Tricep Pushes	1 hr 30 mins 1.5 hrs	30 reps 1 round 50 reps
DAY 3	• Stretching & warm-up • Tempo-run 3 miles • Chest and shoulders	20 min 1,.5 hrs 2 hrs.	5 times 1 round 20 reps
DAY 4	• Legs and cardio • Easy run 3 miles • Wall Tricep Pushes	1 hr 30 mins 1.5 hrs	30 reps 1 round 50 reps
DAY 5	• Stretching & warm-up • Tempo-run 3 miles • Chest and shoulders	20 min 1,.5 hrs 2 hrs.	5 times 1 round 20 reps

WEEKLY FITNESS TRACKER

DATE

CURRENT WEIGHT

	DURATION	ACTIVITY
S		
M		
T		
W		
TH		
F		
S		

AFFIRMATIONS

I am

MON
_____
_____

TUE
_____
_____

WED
_____
_____

THU
_____
_____

FRI
_____
_____

SAT
_____
_____

SUN
_____
_____

DATE

Reflection

date:

_____

_____

_____

_____

_____

_____

_____

_____

_____

_____

_____

_____

_____

_____

_____

_____

_____

_____

_____

_____

Weekly Goal Planner

The Goal:

The Strategy:

Steps to Take:

-
-
-
-
-
-

Other Notes

List Your #4 Goal

When do you think it will be completed?

Did you accomplish this goal?

Reflection

date:

Do one thing everyday that scares you and do it well.

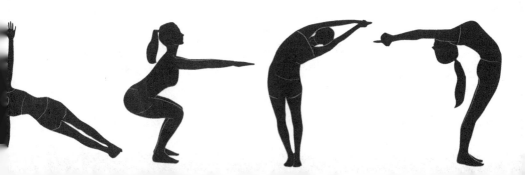

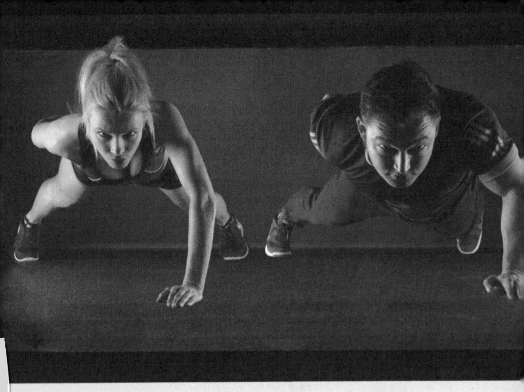

" Workout because you love your self "

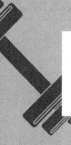

WORK IT!

WORKOUT PLANNER

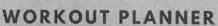

	ACTIVITY	TIME	REPS
DAY 1	• Stretching & warm-up • Tempo-run 3 miles • Chest and shoulders	20 min 1,.5 hrs 2 hrs.	5 times 1 round 20 reps
DAY 2	• Legs and cardio • Easy run 3 miles • Wall Tricep Pushes	1 hr 30 mins 1.5 hrs	30 reps 1 round 50 reps
DAY 3	• Stretching & warm-up • Tempo-run 3 miles • Chest and shoulders	20 min 1,.5 hrs 2 hrs.	5 times 1 round 20 reps
DAY 4	• Legs and cardio • Easy run 3 miles • Wall Tricep Pushes	1 hr 30 mins 1.5 hrs	30 reps 1 round 50 reps
DAY 5	• Stretching & warm-up • Tempo-run 3 miles • Chest and shoulders	20 min 1,.5 hrs 2 hrs.	5 times 1 round 20 reps

WEEKLY FITNESS TRACKER

DATE

CURRENT WEIGHT

	DURATION	ACTIVITY
S		
M		
T		
W		
TH		
F		
S		

AFFIRMATIONS

I am

MON _____
_____

TUE _____
_____

WED _____
_____

THU _____
_____

FRI _____
_____

SAT _____
_____

SUN _____
_____

DATE _____

Weekly Goal Planner

The Goal:

The Strategy:

Steps to Take:

- [ ]
- [ ]
- [ ]
- [ ]
- [ ]
- [ ]

Other Notes

What goal didn't you accomplish?

How do you feel about it?

What can you do differently this week?

Reflection

date:

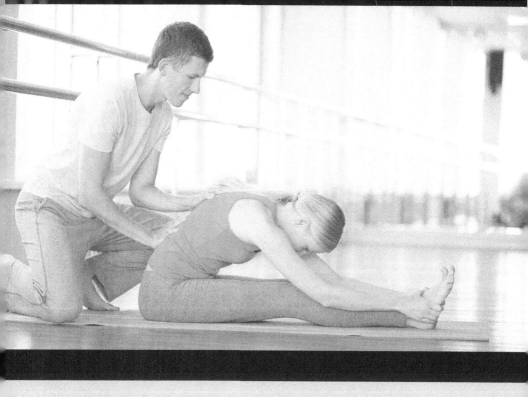

Push harder than yesterday for a different tomorrow

Made in the USA
Middletown, DE
05 October 2023

40277309R00057